To live each day

Stories by people with cancer

Walter Stratford

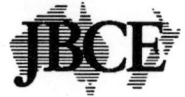

The Joint Board of Christian Education
Melbourne

Published by
THE JOINT BOARD OF CHRISTIAN EDUCATION
65 Oxford Street, Collingwood 3066, Australia

TO LIVE EACH DAY

© Walter Stratford 1995

This publication is copyright. Other than for the purposes and subject to the conditions prescribed under the Copyright Act, no part of it may in any form or by any means (electronic, mechanical, microcopying, photocopying, recording or otherwise) be reproduced, stored in a retrieval system or transmitted without prior written permission from the publisher.

Scripture quotations are from the *Revised Standard Version of the Bible*, copyrighted 1946, 1952, © 1971, 1973 by the Division of Christian Education of the National Council of Churches of Christ in the USA; and from the *New English Bible*, second edition © 1970 by permission of Oxford and Cambridge University Presses.

National Library of Australia
 Cataloguing-in-Publication entry.

Stratford, W. B.
 To live each day: a reflective journey into the lives of people with cancer.

 ISBN: 1 86407 068 4.

 1. Cancer – Patients – Biography. 2. Cancer – Religious aspects – Christianity. 3. Cancer – Patients – Religious life. I. Joint Board of Christian Education. II. Title.

248.86

First printed 1995.

Cover photo by Skjold Photographs
Cover design by Robina Norton
Design by Patricia Baker
Typeset by JBCE in Bodoni Book
Printed by Australian Print Group

JB95/3604

Contents

Acknowledgments 5
Introduction 7
    George 9
    Valda 11
    Graham 17
    Gwen 21
    Moreen 25
    John 28
    Jan 31
    Noel 34
    Marie 40
    Felicity 44
    Jim 50
    Dawn 53
    Myra 56
    Susan 63
    Bob 67
    Betty 72
    Ken 77
Epilogue 80

Acknowledgments

My special thanks to Betty, Bob, Dawn, Felicity, George, Graham, Gwen, Jan, Jim, John, Ken, Marie, Moreen, Myra, Noel, Susan and Valda who told me their stories and who continued to show a keen interest in the progress of the book.

Thanks also to Rosemary who read each segment with a critical eye and to colleagues who encouraged me.

Introduction

This book is about people with cancer. The stories, written by cancer patients, are about their hopes and fears. They write of the shock of learning they have cancer, and of the difficulties they experienced living with their cancer and the treatment they received. Their stories have been interwoven with poetry, Scripture and prayer.

Being told one has cancer is rather like being told one is forsaken. Life for most people is ongoing. It is to be enjoyed and planned for. The new house, new baby, new grandchild are part of the process of life unfolding and we expect that all these things will come to pass in good order. Deep down we know we will eventually die but such an event is rarely part of our planned life.

Suddenly, shatteringly, the plan is changed, truncated, perhaps reduced to nothing and years reduced to days. For many, the psalmist's cry is their cry...

> My God, my God, why hast thou forsaken me
> and art so far from saving me, from heeding my groans?
> O my God, I cry in the day-time but thou dost not answer,
> in the night I cry but get no respite.'
>
> Psalm 22:1-2. (*New English Bible*)

The cry frequently does not elicit an answer but it does allow expression of the anger, despair and grief which well up from the pit of our stomach. It is only after the blaming and guilt and fear have subsided that we can begin to be in touch with the psalmist who says...

> But thou art he who drew me from the womb,
> who laid me at my mother's breast.
> Upon thee was I cast at birth;
> from my mother's womb thou hast been my God.

Be not far from me,
for trouble is near, and I have no helper.

       Psalm 22:9-11. (*New English Bible*)

Now we may begin to live each day, hesitantly at first but with growing confidence and enjoyment of another day of living creatively and lovingly.

George

Christmas is a time of beginnings, a remembering of the birth of a child, of God's coming to be with people.

At such a time, to suddenly discover not beginnings, but endings was a shattering experience for George and no doubt is for many.

Even at that first Christmas, there was the foreshadowing of an end. The baby was born into perilous times and powerful forces were ranged against him from the beginning. God did not come close to people to make their life beautiful. Rather the Word spoke of a different way of living, of new possibilities, of a mystery that lies beyond us but links us to eternity.

This is also a beginning.

One week before Christmas 1992, as preparations for the family celebrations were under way, I became aware of a slight crackling in my upper chest area. My doctor couldn't find anything alarming but ordered an X-ray anyway. The result was to prove to be the most shattering news. I had terminal lung cancer! It is very difficult to describe my feelings at this time.

The realisation that I would leave my family was the most traumatic thought to deal with. Then followed the course of radiotherapy with its side effects and then the chemotherapy sessions which in turn take a toll in strength and resources.

During this time, my mind experienced anguish, bitterness and the inevitable, why me? However, the support of my family, my true friends and the compassion of doctors and staff at the Cancer Care Centre gradually took over my reasoning.

As I approach the completion of my treatment, more and more I realise that each day now is a good day. I do not dwell on my original prognosis of a few months to live but rather trust in a Higher Power to guide me through this dash thing.

A present for Christmas

Not much of a present,
Lord,
this cancer
moving within.

Instead of joy,
anguish!
bitterness!
Why me?
Yet joy I
still find
in those who
love
and care.

Each day,
Lord,
hold my hand
and help me through.

■■■

Hear, O Lord, when I call aloud;
show me favour and answer me.
'Come', my heart has said, 'seek his face'.
I will seek thy face, O Lord;
Do not hide it from me.

Psalm 27:7-9 (*New English Bible*)

■■■

Prayer

God of beginnings and endings, be with us at our beginnings and our endings, and the times in between.

Valda

When we take the time to draw a map of our life, we become aware of many features that at other times we keep tucked away in our memory. On that map, there are high points like the birth of a much wanted child and low points such as the discovery of disease and the death of a loved one. Sometimes, as we look at our map the low points exceed the high points and we wonder why this might be so.

There are times, as Valda says, when events can be shattering. Unexpected news, not being told the full story, others making decisions on our behalf, can be traumatic experiences. These experiences frequently play havoc with our emotions, evoking anger and fear. These responses are natural and need to be allowed to flow freely so that we can find appropriate ways for dealing with our illness.

When we draw maps of our life, we do not always take account of qualities such as strength, loving, caring friends and family. Similarly we tend to neglect our creative resolve in the face of adversity and the spiritual resources which are potentially available to all. A map of these qualities is often rather different from a map of events.

In Valda's story, these facets are interwoven and show a life which, despite adversity, expresses joy and a trust in resources beyond the human.

Valda, her husband and family moved to the Sunshine Coast in 1973 where eventually a beautiful baby daughter was born in 1974. She writes of suffering with mastitis and finding lumps in her breast which culminated in a mastectomy which she found traumatic. She writes, 'I did not give permission for mastectomy and was shattered when matron told me I would have to go back to surgery for removal of my breast'.

Valda writes, 'My operation was followed by a course of radium treatment in Brisbane which made me very sick. During this time, I missed seeing our daughter take her first steps. My mother stayed at our home and once again cared for our baby, whilst my husband, before and after work, cared for our sons and helped with household chores. On arriving home my family were wonderful to me. I prayed constantly and gained strength. One special prayer was "Please, Lord, let me live long enough to raise our children"'.

Problems continued, with her husband becoming ill and further lumps developing for Valda. Her husband was found to have Mesothelioma (cancer caused through asbestos) and even though he had some chemotherapy treatment, he did not respond. At this time, Valda was in need of further surgery for the removal of lumps but also needed to care for her husband.

She writes, 'I prayed for a solution to our problems and was blessed with a phone call from interstate. It was my brother-in-law who insisted that I book myself into hospital. He was on the next plane and cared for our children. He took me to hospital in Nambour and my husband to Chermside the same day.

'After three months of extreme pain, my husband mercifully passed away in January 1981. My family and I were devastated. Our children were aged fifteen, thirteen and six. Our grief was hard to bear. Our elder son appeared to grow up quickly and began to take some responsibility in caring for myself, his brother and sister. We became closer always talking over any problems. Friends drove me to the shops once a week, as I could not carry heavy loads, and during this time I secured my driver's licence and found it was great being able to get my own shopping and take the children to school and other functions.'

After her mother's death, Valda was able to enjoy a holiday through the generosity of a neighbour. Other operations followed and Valda developed an interest in diet and in fitness classes.

She says, 'However, too many arm exercises were given and my arm became very swollen and sore. I was told by a doctor that nothing could be done to help the situation. I was later to find that this was not so and became a patient at the Wesley Hospital's Lymphoedema Clinic. Through hand massage and treatment on a pressure pump, with subsequent bandaging, my condition was soon under control. I massage the lymphatic areas of my body each day and do special exercises'.

Further operations helped her to remain well for a time but eventually she was referred to an oncologist who discovered problems in her lungs. With suitable medication, her lungs responded.

Valda takes up the story again. 'Some time later, however, I developed thirteen lumps across my mastectomy cut. A discussion was held with my oncologist and radiologist who both agreed I could not at this stage have radium as the area to be treated was extensive. I therefore had no alternative but to commence chemotherapy. This treatment made me very sick but thankfully I did not lose my hair. After several treatments, the lumps became smaller and some receded making it possible to hit the larger ones with radium. A product named *Ondansetron* became available which stopped the vomiting occurring after chemotherapy and, although not feeling the best for a few days after treatment, I am able to cope with the situation and lead a busy life.

'I became interested in meditation and became aware of the healing power within me. I have met people who, having been given a death sentence for cancer by their doctor, became well after regular meditation. I believe there are many factors in maintaining good health. I would list faith as a prime factor, followed by expert medical attention, a good balanced diet, a positive attitude, meditation, exercise, and rest when necessary. Love plays an important part. Love for family, friends and those around us and learning to forgive and not harbour grudges. Also it is advisable to avoid stressful situations wherever possible.

'In October 1991, whilst holidaying on the Gold Coast, I suddenly developed stomach pains during a musical show and for several days suffered severe vomiting and on being sent for stomach X-rays and then to a specialist, was immediately admitted to hospital. An operation revealed a hernia which had ruptured my bowel and was gangrenous. A part of the bowel was removed. My family were told there was a thirty-five percent mortality rate with this kind of operation. I was fed through a tube with special exotic fruits and was told my immune system was lowered due to the severe diet I had been following. As a result, my blood sugar level rose and had to be checked every four hours. As it was too high I was then given insulin. I was also given two blood transfusions.

'One week after my operation, I developed an infection causing swelling to the whole of my body. I was desperately ill and it became apparent to me that this time I might not survive. I prayed constantly, especially on the hour, which got me through the long sleepless nights. I prayed to the Lord saying, "I am willing to fight to get well but it is up to you – it is in your hands". I stopped worrying and was at peace, feeling whichever way things went it was OK by me. I believe the Lord, hearing my prayer, gradually brought back my strength and helped me to recover.

'I would like to share an article from the book *God at Eventide* with which I was very impressed.

The war within

> And he was dumb because he believed not.
> There is a physical correspondence to faith and to doubt.
> Especially is this so among those who would serve me.
> For unlike others, they are not controlled
> by the law of physical success or failure, but are under the direct control of the laws of my Kingdom.
>
> So, in many cases, you may note good health
> in one ignorant of Me and ill health
> in one of My followers, until he has learned

the full control of the physical by the Spiritual.
In his case the warring of physical and Spiritual
may cause physical ill health, or unrest.
So do not fret about the physical side,
aim increasingly at control by My Spirit.

(Reprinted from A. J. Russell (ed.), *God at Eventide*, Daystar, Fortitude Valley, 1981.)

'I have had six courses of radium treatment, the last five free from nausea. My radiologist warned the last couple of times that, due to the amount of treatment I had already received, there was a possibility I may develop an ulcer. I prayed throughout both treatments asking to be spared from ulcers or severe burns. I was free from ulcers, only slight burning occurred in the first instance and my skin remained completely normal following my last treatment.

'Our two sons are now happily married and our daughter is eighteen and a great comfort to me. The Lord has thankfully answered my prayer made so many years ago after my mastectomy and has supported me at all times. My illness has made me more aware of the suffering of others and given me confidence in discussing and sharing their problems. I feel, in this way, I have been truly blessed.'

■■■

Lumps

Will I ever be free
from lumps?

The doctor said,
'cut this!
remove that!
Radiotherapy!
Chemotherapy!'
Will I ever be free
from lumps?
I can put up
with lumps
Lord,
as long as you
stay close
and hold my hand.

■ ■ ■

The Lord is my light and my salvation;
whom shall I fear?
The Lord is the stronghold of my life;
of whom shall I be afraid?
                Psalm 27:1 (*Revised Standard Version of the Bible*)

■ ■ ■

Prayer

**God of rough and smooth places,
hold my hand and lift me when I stumble.**

Graham

When life becomes for us an exciting, fulfilling adventure, interwoven with love and friendship, then we are really blessed. When, faced by a disease which may take away that life sooner than we anticipated, we can still find pleasure and fulfilment, we are truly blessed.

Life is, for many, not like this and yet still there is frequently a sense of blessing, a sense of the presence of God.

Life surrounds us with mystery. There is so much in it that we do not understand. Perhaps we are not meant to understand the details of life so much as to live. Each day is precious and can be special for each of us.

Living, content with mystery, is to experience something of the mystery of God and in this experience be blessed.

I have had a wonderful life, and although my circumstances have changed dramatically in recent years, I am still enjoying a wonderful life.

My fortune began with my choice of parents, for they strove to give me the love and every social and educational opportunity that a child needs. My childhood began in New Guinea and, interrupted by the war, continued into youth and young adulthood in Queensland. My exceptional enjoyment of life was catalysed by loyal and exciting friends, a boat to play with on the river, a bike to explore the roads, many sporting activities and membership of scouts and YMCA.

My very best friend became my wife Florence, with whom I have now shared my life for over thirty years. We raised a family of four, whom we have guided to productive adult lives. An intelligent and Christian woman, Florence has supported me in all my endeavours, just as I have tried to support her. Since I was diagnosed with an aggressive and incurable cancer, she has redoubled her efforts to care for me and together with a certain amount of invaluable medical help, we have kept me in much better physical condition than anybody dared to expect.

Study interfered with the more rewarding activities I pursued as a youth and young adult, but, probably with a good deal of divine intervention, I managed to graduate from university. A career as an agricultural scientist offered me a highly diversified, challenging and engrossing occupation and allowed me to exploit my deep love of the land and nature. Agricultural patrols on foot to serve the villagers in the rugged mountains, coastal areas and islands of the Huon Peninsula in New Guinea gave me the privilege of experiencing the local cultures at first hand.

Agricultural research in Papua New Guinea and Queensland acquainted me closely with such diverse fields as wet tropical farming systems, soils, plant nutrition, pasture establishment, fruit and vegetable production, and even the relationship between flying foxes and fruit production. I diversified my fields of expertise by studying agricultural extension, allowing me to promulgate farming knowledge more effectively to Queensland's horticultural growers.

But diagnosis of a terminal cancer cut my career disappointingly short, leaving uncompleted several of my exciting projects, including support for potential new horticultural industries for Queensland.

Now I concentrate on the business of living – not dying. Florence's love, the companionship of family and friends, good music, informative reading, my happy memories and regular interesting activities, all linked by God's loving Spirit, combine to give me a wholly fulfilled lifestyle. In all I have done throughout my life, I have tried to exemplify my spiritual beliefs and Christian values, first imparted to me by my parents. These same principles are continuing to sustain me now. I don't fear dying – my life has already been fulfilled. My only regret will be leaving Florence alone, and I pray that somehow, she will receive the same loving support that she has given me.

■■■

Within my life

Within my life
much has been
accomplished.
Life has been for me
a thing of joy
achieving much,
yet loving simple things.

Now,
with loving wife,
I live more
quietly.
Adventuring no more.

Now reflections
are my adventuring,
as in my quietness
I find love,
fulfilment,
and a sense
of presence;
of mystery.

■■■

I waited patiently for the Lord;
he inclined to me and heard my cry.
He drew me up from the desolate pit,
out of the miry bog,
and set my feet upon a rock,
making my steps secure.
Psalm 40:1-2 (Revised Standard Version of the Bible)

Prayer

God of mystery, bless us with contentment.

Gwen

Someone once said to me, 'Being told you have cancer is like being hit with a club'. I guess that many have walked out of a doctor's surgery in a haze, disbelieving, yet knowing deep down that what they have been told is true.

It is natural, and I believe helpful, in the early days to disbelieve. It's as if our mind needs time to catch up with what we've heard. Once it has caught up, we are able to deal with the problem.

Dealing with the problem can open our eyes to a world we never realised existed. We see our surroundings with a new clarity and begin to find wonders in what once was mundane.

Life can be marvellous and easy, despite pain, despite medication, despite the presence within.

The Spirit of God is also a presence within.

When my GP told me there could be a serious problem with some blood test results and mentioned a type of cancer, I couldn't believe it was happening to me. On leaving the clinic, I walked a long distance to a shopping complex. I felt I was walking well above the footpath, walking through a haze, not concentrating, separate from the rest of the world.

Days passed and I didn't tell anyone for a few weeks because I still thought there may be a mistake with the blood tests and I felt if I put my worries into words they would begin to seem more real and I guess I didn't want to accept that. This is what is termed denial, I suppose.

I didn't feel sick or have any pain. I'd only had the blood tests to check on a bit of tiredness. Eventually my specialist confirmed my condition. I still smiled and felt it couldn't be true. I know it is, of course, and I thank the Lord for sending me along for the blood tests as my cancer was caught in early stages.

After my first visit to my specialist which confirmed my GP's opinion, it still took me a long time to believe it was all happening. I wasn't frightened and I don't think I ever have been. But when you realise your life span had probably been shortened, or has it? Maybe I would have had a road accident or a heart attack even sooner; no one knows what is ahead of them.

Certainly life takes on a different meaning and you realise that the sun and the moon rise and set each day, the sky seems more blue and the grass greener. Flowers are brighter colours – even the veins on the leaves, the shapes, the drops of rain look like diamonds. All things you may have not even bothered to notice before make you feel life can still be beautiful.

That was all nearly two years ago. Since then I have had pain and I've been sick. The days leading up to my first chemotherapy were full of tension. Will I be sick? Will I lose my hair? I wasn't sick but I did lose my hair. That to me was awful but taught me I was probably vain.

My first visit to the Day Care Centre was a particularly scary day. I had all sorts of tests in readiness for the first chemotherapy. I felt so lonely walking through the treatment room to be weighed and measured. I felt that all the patients who were having chemo were watching me and maybe feeling sorry for me. I know now as I sit there myself, I don't take a lot of notice of the other patients but when I do see someone coming through for the first time I wonder if they are feeling the way I did. I feel sorry for them and hope my thoughts get to them and give them encouragement. Of course once we've been there a few times and have learned the procedures and talked to the very caring staff, nothing is frightening anymore.

I've had a spell in hospital with fractured bones, followed by radiotherapy. This was frightening first time only because it's the beginning of another unknown treatment, but it didn't hurt a bit and the staff were always so encouraging.

At present I'm feeling quite well, helped by the loving care of my family, specialist and nursing staff. I know I've got a long way to go. I was born in 1925 and taught to say my prayers from the time I could talk. Always starting with

> Now I lay me down to sleep,
> I pray thee, Lord, my soul to keep.
> If I should die before I wake,
> I pray thee, Lord, my soul to take.

I remember when I was very young, I didn't like the idea of 'dying before I wake'. Now I feel safe when I say that prayer. Yes, I still say it.

■■■

You have cancer

You have cancer
the doctor said.

Dazed,
I walked as if
my feet
did not belong to me
A mistake perhaps?
Could it really
happen to me?

But then I thought
of Sun and Stars
of sky blues
and grass greens,
diamond droplets
of rain
glistening with new beauty,
and knew again
the presence
of the keeper
of souls.

■ ■ ■

> In the beginning was the Word, and the Word was with God and the Word was God. He was in the beginning with God; all things were made through him, and without him was not anything made that was made....
> And the Word became flesh...
>
> John 1:1-5, 14 (*Revised Standard Version of the Bible*)

■ ■ ■

Prayer

Keeper of souls, hold me close to your heart.

Moreen

Tiredness seems inevitably to be a by-product of cancer. Chemo and radiotherapy may leave the body drained of energy. As blood deteriorates, the body becomes more listless because the oxygen intake has lessened. A blood transfusion can, and usually does, make a world of difference for a time.

Coping with life and the demands of family can be particularly tiring when coping with cancer at the same time.

Then there is the deep down tiredness that settles within us as life becomes more and more difficult and we begin to move towards dying. Moreen says in her story, 'I'm so tired now'. Her words suggest that for her, this is a tiredness which leads into eternal sleep.

Such a sleep as this is frequently something we fear, but sleep we must eventually. Perhaps the deep down tiredness is God's way of reminding us of our need to sleep. Perhaps it also suggests to us that even in the deepest of sleeps – death itself – God is present and secures us in God's presence.

It is now eighteen months since I found out I had cancer. I find it hard to recall my feelings but know in later months I have come to terms with it. Reading from the experience of others who have had to cope, relating to their feelings of depression and fear of how the end will go. Trying to tell God exactly how I felt and a lot of resting in the prayers of others who have been praying for me has meant a lot. Now I look forward to being with my saviour who has been very precious to me throughout my life.

People of all denominations have been very kind and within everyone there appears to be a faith that shines in times of crisis. I do sincerely praise God for people and that he knows what is ahead and pray for faith to keep trusting whatever. I pray for those who do pastoral care work and all volunteers. One only has to lift one's feeling to God and that is prayer.

Being aware somewhat of what may lie ahead, I sometimes fear the symptoms, especially fear of breathing problems, but have learnt to trust and to leave it to the One who knows it all. So, together with the prayers of so many lovely people, I seek to rest in him. It is not always easy but I have encouragement from others who have learnt to cope, taking a day at a time. I would like the time I have left to be a witness to him who has meant much to me throughout my lifetime and to my family.

Praise God for his many, many blessings – especially family, friends and all who volunteer to help. God is really so good.

I feel this is a very poor effort but I am so tired and do not concentrate as I used to.

■■■

I'm tired

God
I'm tired!
Yet still I seek
to know your will.

Throughout my life
I have been blessed
through
many friends
whose faith
has been a light
to me.

> As my life here
> draws to a close,
> hold my hand
> and still my fears
> Draw me quietly
> into your presence.

■ ■ ■

Praise the Lord!
How good it is to sing praises
to our God;
for he is gracious...
>> Psalm 147:1 (*Revised Standard Version of the Bible*)

■ ■ ■

Prayer

**O God who never sleeps,
be with me in my sleeping
and waken me into your presence.**

John

Being told you have cancer and that a major operation is required immediately is a traumatic experience. As John notes, one has to prepare one's own mental outlook about the disease, inform family and get ready for an operation virtually all at the same time.

Added to all this, finding on waking up that one has to carry an external apparatus to collect body wastes means that in a very short space of time one needs to make major mental and emotional changes and accept major body changes as well. Yet somehow people find, as John did, the resources to cope with these rather extreme circumstances and emerge relatively unscathed. Certainly one answer as to how people are able to do this lies in the support of groups and individuals, of organisations and of family. Perhaps there is also an unrecognised resource which rests within us and which some call the Spirit of God. Perhaps the Spirit works a little like a slow release fertiliser in a garden, releasing energy as it is needed.

July the 7th was the day I had a colonoscopy and the day the doctor informed me I had a large tumour in my bowel and an operation was required. July the 10th I was operated on. I must confess that in the time between the 7th and 10th there were more than a few tears shed as I found that informing my family of my sickness was harder than my accepting that I had cancer.

To my surprise, I did not say 'why me?' as I had a suspicion I had cancer, but that did not make it easier to accept. My first thoughts were I must be strong for my family and have a positive outlook. I have cancer and it won't go away by feeling sorry for myself.

During the operation it was found that I required a colostomy which I found on awaking from the operation 'quite a shock' as I didn't know how I would handle this new problem. After a few days and with support of my family and the nursing staff, I discovered it wasn't much of a problem after all.

We received support from the Queensland Cancer Fund and the Queensland Colostomy Association. Four months after the operation, my bowel had recovered well enough so the colostomy was reversed and the bowel rejoined. This also caused a few problems but nothing that I could not overcome.

I needed thirty sessions of radiation and fifty-two of chemotherapy. At the time of writing, I am thirty-four weeks into the chemotherapy. At the fifty-second, my last dose of chemo (I pray), we will be having a big celebration. I am coping very well with the chemo and have started back to full time employment six months after the operation.

To finish off, my outlook is this: I have cancer and feeling sorry won't cure it. There are people and groups who will give help; all that is required is for you to ask for it. Don't keep things bottled up within yourself. Family support is very important. Keep a positive outlook; you will always find someone else who is worse off than yourself. One can only look to the future and hope and pray that everything will turn out OK.

PS My age at the time of writing is fifty-four years.

■■■

7 July

On this day the doctor
said,
'Cancer'.
'Operation'.

And I,
with tears,
must tell my family

> of this thing
> that lurked within;
> silently threatening.
>
> But now,
> enfolded by loving family,
> upheld by friends and
> strangers
> I look in hope
> towards
> a day of celebration!

■■■

I lift up my eyes to the hills
from where will my help come?
My help comes from the Lord,
who made heaven and earth.
Psalm 121:1-2 (Revised Standard Version of the Bible)

■■■

Prayer

**God of fears and tears,
help us to know your presence within
as love and new life,
spreading energy that stems the fears
and heals the tears.**

Jan

It is often a worry to us when we feel unwell and don't seem to be able to find a cause. A diagnosis, even when its name is cancer, can be, as it was for Jan, a release from the worry. When we have found the cause of our problem we can get on with treating it and thus feel that something positive is being done.

As we progress through that treatment, of course, other feelings emerge and will need to be dealt with. Perhaps the important thing about dealing with our emotions is that we don't try to do it all at once. If we expect to lump all our emotions together and then sort them out, we may be very disappointed. It is more realistic to try and resolve them one at a time.

Jan found others to help her in this process. It is important for each one of us to seek the support of groups and individuals and also to be aware when we may need more specialised help.

My first reaction when I heard I had a tumour and needed an operation was one of relief. The cause of my low blood count and not feeling well had been found.

That the tumour was malignant in answer to my asking did not particularly concern me. My doctor explained very carefully the procedure and the outcome for the future and I had full confidence in what he told me.

The weekly treatment I have had for the last nine months has had its ups and downs but on the whole I feel I have coped pretty well. I must admit I am counting down the last weeks to the finish of treatment.

What surprised me was that, after six months, I found myself in a situation where I had emotional and relationships issues to come to terms with. The fact that I had had cancer (and I stress *had*) was always positive and no misgivings about the future were even thought of by me. However, the issues that caused me anger and confusion were probably more important than the physical side which had been the most prominent issue and the one most discussed. It has taken time and some grieving to sort out where I was, what I am and how to resolve the concerns. I sought help with this and learnt that everyone having had a life threatening experience such as facing cancer, will have feelings and concerns to work through.

Different things trigger off issues for each person. My recent involvement with the Positive Attitude to Cancer Treatment(PACT) program has been very beneficial. The support of the staff at the Day Centre and the open and caring environment has helped me to face each treatment day.

■■■

Relief

When my doctor
said to me
you have a tumour,
I felt
relief.
For now
I could begin to live
is such a way
that healing
might find a place
in me.

> With help of friends,
> anger and
> confusion
> have found
> their proper place
> within,
> and left me space
> to find my way
> each day.

■ ■ ■

Hear my cry, O God,
listen to my prayer;
from the end of the earth
I call to thee,
when my heart is faint.
> Psalm 61:1-2 (*Revised Standard Version of the Bible*)

■ ■ ■

Prayer

**God of illness and health,
lead me through my painful emotions
to a place of understanding.**

Noel

> Many people have talked to me about fighting their cancer and they have indeed waged war on the disease with medicines, radiotherapy and a great deal of determination. I have often wondered, however, as I have listened to people, whether there might be a different way of dealing with cancerous cells and have talked at times of flowing with life and of developing an inner stillness.
>
> Noel's story tells of his rediscovery of inner being and the need to be in touch with his inner self. Perhaps from his reflections we can learn some new ways of continuing life's journey even with cancer, and more importantly, begin to touch our inner self, that place where the Spirit dwells. Perhaps when we make contact with the Spirit, energy will be released and flow through our body in a gentle healing fashion and begin to make us new. Perhaps you also can reflect on your cancer as a gift and use it accordingly.

As a pastor who had frequently ministered to families in which cancer was present, present to the point of death, I had often reflected that one of the blessings of cancer was that it gives time to review life, to set new goals, to tidy up matters, to prepare for death. When I had to face the fact that I had cancer, these sentiments became more than an intellectual response; they became the existential centre of my being. How was I to approach my cancer as a gift, an opportunity, a freedom, a new chance!

From my childhood I had embraced optimism, faith, hope as the basic orientation of my life, even though I had seen much pain and suffering and apparent hopelessness in many others and in my study of society, and not surprisingly I had lived with depression requiring medical assistance for many years. Still my fundamental belief and message whenever I found a pulpit or a lecture theatre was: 'Keep hope alive, believe things can be changed'.

When I first was diagnosed as having bowel cancer, I had one night of fear, but it seemed that facing that fear opened the way for healing and hope to take over my consciousness. Indeed, I said to many at the time, healing began once the diagnosis was known; healing in many senses, especially healing of relationships and the harm of being 'driven' in my work habits. Indeed I came to understand the removal of my cancerous tumour as a cleansing of 'the messiness' of recent years and as a new beginning, not only with my new bowel, but in a wider, more profound sense as well. In a true sense, I interpret the surgery as sacramental, an outward sign of an inward grace.

My brief stay in hospital was a beautiful gift, a 'high', a peak experience indeed. Many things became clear. I need have no delusions; life is uncertain and I was living in the end times when it is possible to see more clearly what matters most.

I saw clearly why my cancer developed. In fact, I didn't go through a stage of 'why me?'. I could see ample reason why me! (Though, later, I did have some anger, feeling 'if only...' 'why now, why not later?') It is not important that I share the reasons for my cancer developing but I believe it is important to try to identify the psychosomatic dimensions of the disease and deal with them as far as possible.

I found myself freely expressing to visitors and friends who may not have shared Christian faith, that God had touched me, that this was a remarkable advent (for it was December), and that Jesus' words 'I have come that you might have life in all its fullness' took on renewed power fo me. I became profoundly aware that this experience was a gift to renew ministry, but that the beginning of that ministry was to myself.

Like many before me, I read and re-read the range of literature on treatment and the amazing stories of recovery, while becoming unquestionably aware that cancer is potent to the point of death again and again, though not always. I had to face the medical facts: my condition was such that I had a greater than fifty percent chance of recurrence within the next four to five years and that when, or if, the cancer recurred, I would be into the harsh, painful fight which, in orthodox medical terms, is very unlikely to result in remission.

My quest for knowledge gave me, and those close to me, a quantitative leap in understanding the body, disease and medicine. I sought a package of therapy and therapists which would leave me responsible for the changes in my life and path to recovery. There is no point in laying out my chosen recipe: it may not prove effective at the survival level, and furthermore I believe each individual must find their own path. However, I have come to the conclusion that rest, relaxation and meditation (and, with them, freedom from stress) are vital.

Above all, I decided to trust my body and its recuperative power and to listen to and care for my body much more than I had in the past. I resolved also that a closer journey with my God (the journey inward) would become central in the next stage of my life. I wrote to friends at the time: 'Obviously the cancer and subsequent recuperation is a gift to enable me to review my vocations of ministry, teaching and public witness'.

One of the critical realisations I had to confront in the post-operative stage was how to conceptualise and visualise the so-called 'fight' with cancer. I learnt that the tumour and any cancer seedlings or 'hot spots' still active in my body, are cells of my tissue, not foreign to my body but of me, even though they are rogue cells. Eradicating cancer and fighting cancer may be a misdirected understanding. While it cannot be denied that every cancer patient and society addressing this health problem are engaged in a fight and a struggle, it seemed to me that the body required gentleness in the process of learning to live with, manage, eradicate and integrate, the potential for cancer that is within me.

It struck me as a bit like Jung's interpretation of coming to terms with the shadow side within me. Though I am not comfortable with imagery that sets up a war within me, I seek an 'armoury' of measures that are primarily pro-life measures, and, in that sense, anti-cancer.

My tendency to academic reflection posed meaning-of-life questions at another level which I am bound to pursue. Cancer poses such a challenge to medical science that it cannot be dealt with merely scientifically. It pushes us to the converging boundary of philosophy (and/or religion) and science. It invites us to question traditional, western, rationalistic and dualistic paradigms, and to explore the wisdom of Eastern and earth religions in their emphasis on a wholistic world view, involving the uniting of mind and body.

In other words, the issue is a new interaction which does not reject Western technocratic accomplishments altogether but which critically subjects them to a new wisdom that is generally an old wisdom found in ancient and Aboriginal cultures and in the mystic tradition of Judaism and Christianity.

The journey into the land of uncertainty is exciting, giving special joy to each day. I believe it will focus my energies much more creatively. Already it has led me to wonderful resources in books, in music, in people – actually I sit here writing this in the midst of a rainforest, at peace. Stillness, prayerfulness, meditation, contemplation – whatever name you use, I now see is not the added boost to busy lives or the refuge when we are exhausted, but the very centrepoint, the essential out of which wholesome living derives.

One of those persons I have met because of the cancer is a doctor who summarised for me the challenging truth that lies before me, and all of us. It is the challenge to wholeness, a wholeness which combines a readiness to live and a readiness to die. And he reminded me that 'wholeness' derives from an ancient Anglo-Saxon word that has given us the term 'healing' and also 'holiness'. The journey to healing, wholeness and holiness in made on the one path.

■■■

The gift

God gave me a gift!
Tho' some
would not think it so.

This gift
has come to me as
cleansing,
and as
opportunity
to explore my life
again.

To seek wisdom
in the wisdom of
the land,
and of ancient people.
To find again
that which is
the centrepoint of life.

With this gift, Lord,
help me to know
my life
and my death.

Walk with me!

■■■

God is our refuge and strength
a very present help in trouble.
Therefore we will not fear though
the earth should change,
though the mountains shake in
the heart of the sea;
though its waters roar and foam,
though the mountains tremble
with its tumult.
>> Psalm 46:1-3 *(Revised Standard Version of the Bible)*

■■■

Prayer

Giver of gifts,
life and death are both gifts from you.
As we take hold of our gift,
grant us the wisdom to know your constant presence.

Marie

Many like Marie find a great deal of help in their illness through reading their holy books. Marie is an avowed Christian and committed, as she says, to daily reading and searching the Scriptures. Similarly, others find strength in the Koran, or the writings of the Buddha, and so on, while others gain their strength from philosophers and other wisdom writers. Attending to the things that unfold for us from our readings, is a way of focusing on the mysteries and wisdom that give us strength.

Marie says that she is a very positive person and has committed herself to remain this way. She uses her day in such a way as to help herself to remain positive and strong. Not all of us have such a determination and being strong all the time can leave us very vulnerable if our condition suddenly changes. There need to be times when we can permit ourselves to be less than strong.

The other side of active seeking is an awareness of stillness, of being able to enter our inner space and find quietness. It is as important *to be*, as it is *to do*. In simply *being* from time to time, the mystery to which we give a variety of names, may have an opportunity to steal into the cracks and corners of our body, bringing knowledge of life and peace.

In October 1988, I was told I had breast cancer and that I would require surgery to remove my left breast. I accepted the fact that this would happen and then could concentrate on getting well again. I have always been a positive person and my faith is very strong.

Positive people are helpful because they want life and living and positive people help me through Scripture and prayer. Anything of God is helpful for me. One book I have found particularly helpful is titled *Scriptural Keys for Kingdom Living*.

It is important for me that there be no negative feelings because this allows Satan to get a foothold. For me, it is important to keep Satan out.

Important words of Scripture to which I cling include the following:

> I shall not die but live
> to proclaim the works of the Lord.
> Psalm 118:17

> He took away our illnesses and lifted our diseases from us. Matthew 8:17

> The thief comes only to steal, to kill, to destroy; I have come that you may have life, and may have it in all its fullness. John 10:10

> In his own person he carried our sins to the gibbet, so that we might cease to live for sin and begin to live for righteousness. 1 Peter 2:24

I have a notebook of references which I cling to and refer to daily. So everyday I seek to bind Satan and toss him out. When I do this I feel peace.

Physically, I may at times feel pain and at times this makes me feel down but I get help from positive people and from prayer. I try not to have downers and I don't have as many now that I more intentionally read the Bible to find God's Word.

Emotionally, I seek to keep everything on an even keel and in fact do not class myself as being sick.

Spiritually, I feel very strong as I read God's Word and pray. This gives me strength.

■ ■ ■

Each day

Each day
I read God's Word,
and find
in there
strength for my journey.

To keep my mind
on God
is my desire.
To follow God's direction
is my need.

This takes my time,
and yet
I know deep down,
that I must also
be still
and let God in
to my inner room.

To enter there
with God
is to find
peace.

■■■

The Lord is my rock, and my fortress,
and my deliverer,
my God, my rock, in whom I take refuge,
my shield, and the horn of my salvation.
     Psalm 18:2 (*Revised Standard Version of the Bible*)

■■■

Prayer

God of strength and courage,
help us in our life battles to remember
that you are also mystery and stillness.

Felicity

Change is inevitable as we journey through life. Our body grows older, friendships come and go. Many of us, like Felicity, move house and have to find our way into a new community.

Perhaps the most traumatic change of all is the discovery that we or a loved one has developed a terminal illness. Each one of us has to find our own way of coming to terms with this change. If a spouse cannot or will not share feelings at this time, then this time of illness can be very difficult for both people.

Felicity writes of her husband's inability to talk to her or the rest of the family. This was a major problem for her and she was angry at being excluded from her husband's dying.

Her story suggests that sharing in the dying process is supremely important. It allows grief to be shared and explored at the time of parting and also gives time for appropriate goodbyes.

It is just over two and a half years since my husband's death. He died in November 1991 just five days short of our twenty-ninth anniversary. As I had known him since I was eight years old, his death left rather a large gap in my life.

Our three children, all adult, were no longer living at home and Rod had just changed careers at the age of fifty-two. With this change we had two shifts in eighteen months; from Toowoomba, where we had lived for twenty years, to Brisbane where we had grown up and I hoped would never live again. From there we moved to Atherton where I had never even thought of living.

I do not move easily and being at that age in a woman's life where change is inevitable and trying to cope with the empty nest syndrome, this move was particularly traumatic. However, to Atherton we went and I spent nine of the happiest months of my life there. It was cut short however as Rod was diagnosed with cancer of the stomach and we returned to Brisbane for surgery and further treatment.

It was a difficult time. His illness became a barrier between us as his struggle to beat the disease became his sole aim. I felt excluded from his life except as cook and chauffeur and in those long weeks we shared very little, even sleeping in separate rooms. There were no deep and meaningful conversations and certainly no coming to terms with dying and separation. Rod refused to believe he was dying which made it almost impossible to act naturally. We all had to keep up a terrible pretence which, looking back, was probably not the wisest thing to do. But in a sense it was his play and we just had supporting roles.

After he died and reality set in, I was so angry that he had denied us the opportunity to be honest. I remember about a week later that the light bulb in our bedroom needed changing – a job he had always done – and as I stood in the middle of our bed with my arms stretched up I screamed in frustration and absolute rage. I tend to live life on a fairly even keel so this was totally out of character but I did feel better afterwards. It's a funny thing about anger though, you don't always know it's there. There have been two occasions since then when I have discovered a well of anger that, when given the right circumstances, surfaced and shocked me.

Both discoveries were at spiritual retreats. The first I had come to as part of the kitchen team to serve others, and I had a ball until the last afternoon when I was sitting behind some married couples in chapel and their closeness and togetherness produced such resentment, jealously and anger that I felt suffocated and finally ended in tears. It was accentuated by self-pity and I wallowed in it! However it was not without value and I was able to talk about it with a loving team member and work it through.

The second occasion was in December 1993. During this retreat, we were asked to consider the passage of Scripture where Jesus is asked to go to his friend Lazarus who was very ill. He purposely delays the visit and Lazarus has been dead for three days before Jesus finally arrives. His sisters are bereft and tell Jesus it wouldn't have happened if he'd been there. To their amazement Jesus asks for the tomb to be opened and calls to Lazarus to come out.

I thought about this family waiting for their friend to turn up and how they must have felt when Lazarus' special friend didn't come. I did not consciously associate this with my situation but I got so angry at God that I wrote 'Who does God think he is – playing God with people's lives!' Ridiculous? Of course. Irrational? Totally.

There is a term in Scripture that God uses of himself – 'I am who I am'. I understand it to mean that God exists and no explanation of his actions is necessary. That was my conclusion and accepting that brought peace. I learned that God wants my trust whatever the circumstances and that he is big enough to cope with my rage. I cannot change the circumstances of my husband's death so it becomes a pointless exercise to wish things had happened differently

I have come to the realisation that life belongs to the living. This in no way reflects on my love for my husband but that part of my life is over. I have come to this point through my Christian belief that everything happens for eventual good, that I will see my husband again, that death is a doorway, that the best is yet to be.

The hospital offers a wonderful grief counselling service and I owe these counsellors my sanity. My church family, friends old and new, have encouraged and loved me, have rung me and taken me out, have written notes and cards which arrived at perfect moments. But, given that support, there are an awful lot of hours when no-one is there and that terrible pain of loneliness sweeps over unexpectedly.

A darling elderly friend, twice widowed, said, 'You know, I still get lonely'. When I asked how long she'd been on her own, she replied, 'Fourteen years'. I was appalled. I remember driving home, telling myself I'd never survive. Fourteen years was unthinkable. A few days later, while out driving, I suddenly realised something wonderful – I don't have to live fourteen years at a time. I am given one day to live, moment by moment, each day new. I may not even have fourteen years left to live!

What freedom that realisation brought! I admit there are times when I am lonely but I do not have to be swamped by that feeling of desolation and that terrible, terrible pain. Perhaps it would be better to say that now I am alone but not necessarily lonely.

In the beginning of my grieving process – and, yes, it is a process – I wept nearly everywhere I went and on nearly everyone I met, including bank tellers, shop assistants, friends, total strangers. I accepted that tears were part of the territory and told them where I was and we would laugh together. I found the book *Good Grief* which I had read some time ago to be very helpful. I was able to recognise that what was happening was normal. I am not saying I have sailed through without falling flat on my face. There have been lots of ups and downs but the biggest aid to my coming to terms with Rod's death had been acceptance. I have never expected him to walk back into my life, nor have I listened for his car, his footsteps or voice.

I have tried to be honest about my feelings and my situation and that has helped others to be honest with me. I found that my anticipation of special events like birthdays and anniversaries was worse than the actual event. There will always be times of sadness. One of these times will be Rod not being present for his daughter's wedding. We speak of Rod quite naturally and I find that others take their cue from this.

I have not shut out experiences that might cause me pain. I have not struggled against feelings that are a normal part of grief. I have accepted professional counselling. I have asked my friends not to guard their conversation because of my presence. I have accepted that I cannot change my circumstances but I can change the way I respond to them. I have accepted that laughter is a gift of healing and I have laughed a lot. I can thank God for the positives and the negatives of each day. I can accept each day as a gift from God and use it the best way I can. I do not have to live tomorrow, just today. I can live my life as a gift to others.

I can choose... I can choose life.

■■■

God, I was angry!

He left me, Lord!
We could not talk;
could not share
our love
and sadness.

God, I was angry
when he died!
How dare he die
like this.

I'm content now, Lord.
The pain of separation
remains.
But now I see
each day,
and know
that I must
live along my journey.
Sometimes lonely,
yet knowing
Your presence.

■■■

Hear my cry, O God, listen to my prayer.
From the end of the earth I call to thee
with fainting heart;
lift me up and set me upon a rock.
For thou hast been my shelter.
          Psalm 61:1-3 *(Revised Standard Version of the Bible)*

■ ■ ■

Prayer

Lord God,
thank you for hearing my anger
and remaining with me.
Stay with me each day
as I make my way along life's path.

Jim

As we have already seen in this book, the message about cancer comes suddenly, shockingly, and with a sense of impending doom. Those first days, as they were for Jim, and seem to be for most, raise many questions and throw our life into turmoil. People cope with these problems in many ways.

Jim, as a committed Christian and a minister in the church, is able to put his trust in God and place himself in God's hands even though this was not an automatic response. To rest in God's strength is one way of tapping the energy of the Spirit and finding a healing.

It comes as a bit of a shock to receive a message during Religious Education class at school that yesterday's X-rays showed bowel cancer and you are wanted back in the hospital that afternoon... And yet it wasn't, for deep down I knew and had known for some time.

Tests and the operation showed it was all through my liver as well and I was given only a short time to live.

How does one cope? The first few days I was too sick to worry about it, but eventually one begins to grapple with it. The trauma of leaving family... Why has this happened to me?... How can I leave the best security for the future for my family?... all sorts of questions come, to be pushed aside and grappled with, bit by bit.

Perhaps the most important was life after death. I preached and believed without doubt 'Jesus saves unto Eternal Life with God the Father'. Now it was being tested in the reality of my living.

Through my relationship with God and the Scriptures, I came to the place of affirming the reality that had always been my situation. Whether I live, I live unto the Lord. Whether I die, I die unto the Lord. Whether I live, therefore, or die, I am the Lord's.

Only in that 'love of God' could, and were, the other questions dealt with. There have been blessings. God has given me time to get affairs and relationships right. Values changed. The supreme issue of life is God in me, and me in God through Christ... and then everything else in place – including cancer!

The support and prayers of my family, friends, and people I've never known has been, and is, a very important strength in coping with leaving this world – for a better one.

'I know in whom I have believed and am persuaded that he is able to keep that which I have committed unto him against that day'.

∎∎∎

A message at school

Today,
boys and girls,
our lesson
is about
the love of God
in Jesus.

A message?
Excuse me, children,
while I attend
to this
caller.

> God,
> where is your love
> now?
> Must I be one
> to carry this
> presence
> within,
> and die before my time?
>
> Lord,
> my time
> is your time.
> My life is yours.
> Take my hand
> and lead me gently.

■ ■ ■

Save me, O God, by thy name,
and vindicate me by thy might.
Hear my prayer, O God;
give ear to the words of my mouth.
> Psalm 54:1-2 (*Revised Standard Version of the Bible*)

■ ■ ■

Prayer

**God of shocks and frights,
take our hand and steady us.
Keep the shocks and frights from overwhelming us.**

Dawn

Having cancer is one thing, being the spouse of a cancer sufferer is quite another. There is considerable trauma in coming to terms with the fact that one's spouse suddenly has a limited time to live.

The pain of watching another going through difficult days is, as Dawn says, deep within us. One might almost call it soul pain somewhere at the centre of our being. Often anger and guilt can also be found in that inner place.

That inner place is also the dwelling place of the Spirit. As we acknowledge the anger, guilt or other emotions as part of our self and not foreign to us, so we can also begin to acknowledge the Spirit in the same way and let Spirit and emotions be together.

Miracles and healing tend to have stereotypes which are more fantasy than reality. Healing can take place, however, even if we are not cured. Dawn and Jim together have found some of this healing in their lives.

Even after the diagnosis from the X-rays, I still couldn't believe how bad things were until the surgeon actually told me he had removed a cancerous lump from Jim's lower bowel and the cancer had already spread right through his liver. My first question was 'How long?' and the reply, 'Two months, maybe two years'.

I managed to thank the doctor, but I was too stunned to think straight as I returned to sit by Jim. He hadn't had to have a bag which was a relief, but he was so sick and weak and sedated, and still in a great deal of pain. The hospital staff were wonderfully gentle and caring. I thought it funny they called him James almost reverently. He had always been my Jim.

God had prepared wonderful saints in Mt Isa to be there for us during Jim's time in hospital and after he was discharged. Our Presbytery Chairman had arranged return air tickets to Brisbane for extended sick leave or whatever. So many opened their hearts and homes for us when we needed them most, during that time and the weeks that followed. We might have been disturbed about some of the church's failings during the many years of full time ministry, but they really came through for us when we needed them most, as have doctors, nursing staff, the Wesley Hospital and the Wesley Medical Centre where Jim goes for regular chemotherapy.

Our loving heavenly Father has provided us with a delightful little home. Family, friends and strangers lovingly and prayerfully support us. I am thankful for this time to come to terms somehow with maybe having to go it alone without Jim. I know the inner peace that only the Holy Spirit gives – the peace Jesus promised us – and I feel my heavenly Father's loving arms about me. Yet there is a pain that is somewhere deep inside as I watch Jim on his 'not so well' days.

I prayed God would make his life a miracle, and he has. Jim looks good. He didn't lose his hair and he mostly enjoys his food and life – and me, too, I hope! I do enjoy him so. We've been fronted up with miracle diets and do-it-yourself type healing. We've struggled with, 'Do we have enough faith to be healed?' and 'If you don't get healed, it's your lack of faith'. It would be wonderful if God healed him, yet I wonder why we're so reluctant to get to heaven when we know it's such a wonderful place. Death and eternity hold no fears for us. It's just I don't want my Jim to suffer. That's the tough part.

I know Jim's relationship with our Lord is such that he'll be O.K... and so will I.

■ ■ ■

God provides

We have found
in this time
love and care.

Doctors,
nurses,
hospitals,
friends and family,
have come to our aid.

The pain within
us both
has found release
in faith,
that God is!

■ ■ ■

Our steps are made firm by the Lord,
when he delights in our way.
though we stumble, we shall not fall headlong.
for the Lord holds us by the hand.
        Psalm 37:23-24 (*Revised Standard Version of the Bible*)

■ ■ ■

Prayer

**God of faith and hope,
lift us out of the pains we bear,
and carry us quietly into your presence.**

Myra

Myra describes her life with cancer in graphic detail. When told she could go home and die or stay in hospital and die, she refused to give in to what she saw as a defeatist attitude and set out to determine her own future rather than leave it in the hands of 'experts'. A number of times she faced delays in diagnosis which became life-threatening and caused much pain.

Perhaps there have been times in our lives when we have experienced delays, for one reason or another, in our finding out what our particular medical problem has been. Such delays can make us very angry as we feel our life at risk because of another's tardiness. Perhaps at these times we wonder whether those who have the knowledge that we do not have, really care. I suspect also that when we have these angry feelings we frequently suppress them as being unworthy. Anger needs to be expressed in creative ways, however, for us to take control of our lives and move on.

Despite all the delays and feelings of helplessness and fear, Myra has developed a faith life which has sustained her and her husband through difficult times.

Myra pays tribute to all who helped and still help her and I expect we could all point to friends and loved ones who sustain us.

Myra mentions two dreams or hallucinations which spoke to her and became significant turning points for her life. Perhaps we could all pay attention to the dreams we have and find in them some powerful new directions for our lives.

As her story unfolds, we are able to see Myra emerging from deep and serious illness into reasonable health and, despite all, to continue to enjoy her life.

About March 1990, I first felt a small lump in my breast. I remember that twelve months previously I had knocked my breast sharply with the handle of a broom. It was sore for days. I wondered if this could have been the cause of the lump and decided to have the doctor investigate it. As I had not had any family, and as the lump was very small, he felt there was no cause for alarm, and no action was taken. A few months later I developed bronchitis very badly and with the constant coughing, cracked a rib which was discovered after an X-ray, The doctor decided the broken rib was because of the coughing.

In August the same year, while we were in Townsville, I was suffering a lot of pain around the rib area and went to the masseur who thought I must have been involved in a car accident as he could feel more than one broken rib and others cracked. He gave me a couple of massages which did give a little relief at the time.

On our return to Toogoom, I went to the doctor again and he immediately ordered a blood test. The test was sent to Brisbane and later that afternoon my doctor telephoned and told me to go to Maryborough Hospital that afternoon. I was admitted but still did not know the result of the test. At Maryborough Hospital, I had tests taken of the lump in the breast and the lump was ultimately removed.

I was in hospital for three weeks and at the end of this time the doctor told me I was riddled with cancer – breasts primary and bones secondary. At this stage, I was told that the blood tests had shown that the calcium level in my blood was high as the cancer was taking the calcium from my bones and this in turn was overtaxing my kidneys.

I was not given any choice or chance of treatment or operation nor referred to any specialist. I could either go home or stay in hospital until the end. For the first time, my husband Noel had to be told the situation. He sat by my bed holding my hand and I told him what the prognosis was. This was something that I had not been prepared to admit to myself, although I had feared for some time that it would be diagnosed as cancer.

Having nursed my mother for five years before she died of the disease, and then having my father die of cancer, and remembering that one grandparent died of cancer that I knew of, naturally gave me a great fear of what the outcome would be. Noel was shocked and as we both sat there comforting each other Noel said, 'They don't know us, darling. We'll beat it'. We both asked the good Lord to help us and had faith in the fact that he would. We both feel that just simply by praying we got so much comfort and had something to hold on to, and this was our faith.

During the next three years, this faith kept both Noel and me not only comforted but able to face the decisions we had to make and those which were made for us. Without this faith, I don't know how we would have faced the future. To this day, we still pray and thank the Lord for his help and comfort without which our life would have been very different. I would like other people, who are without this faith, to know how much I have gained from knowing that through prayer I have not only been comforted but have found the will and ability to go on.

I made the decision to come home from hospital but I don't remember a lot of what happened during the next three months except that I was very ill, in considerable pain and unable to keep down any food I ate. Noel was a wonderful husband and carer during this time. He would even carry me on his back for me to go to the toilet or to bed as he couldn't help me by any other means of carrying because of my cracked and broken ribs. I was very weak. However, we were facing this crisis together, with the help of the Lord.

Early in 1991, my bowel seized up and twice I was admitted to Hervey Bay Hospital to have this cleared. During this time, we were trying to get referred to Brisbane, which we were finding very difficult. The doctors did not see any point in this. I was, virtually, in my own words, thrown on the scrap heap. There was no point in further treatment. I was, however, still fighting for my health and praying that someone would make a different decision about my condition.

Eventually, we got the hospital doctor to ring the Wesley Hospital in Brisbane and speak to the doctor down there about my condition. The Brisbane doctor replied, 'Get that woman down here immediately'. I was on the aerial ambulance next morning with the help of our minister and my family. I was admitted to Wesley Hospital. Although I had countless tests and treatments, they were not clear in my mind. More, I remember the wonderful nursing and the doctors who looked after me with such care.

I was started on chemotherapy and also had radiotherapy on my spine. I was very ill and the doctor had explained the good and the bad effects of the chemotherapy. However, we prayed that the doctors be guided in their decisions regarding my treatment. In retrospect, these prayers were answered. There is no doubt in my mind and Noel's that our prayers and those of other people for me, have helped me both physically and mentally through this most dramatic period of my life. It also helped Noel through this stage of my illness.

I arrived home after about five weeks or so, knowing that I had to return to Brisbane every month for chemotherapy treatment, with chest X-rays and bone scans every six months. All up, I had lost five stone through all this. Luckily I could afford to lose weight. All through this period, I never lost my sense of humour or my fighting spirit, and this gave me a feeling of normality. Each time I return now for chemo, the doctor, when he sees me, shakes his head in wonder and says, 'Myra, you are unbelievable'.

I had only been home a few weeks when I became very ill, and, with the help of a very kind friend, Noel rushed me through to Nambour where I was taken the rest of the way by ambulance to Wesley Hospital where it was diagnosed that I had double pneumonia. After all, I was very weak and had no resistance because of the constant chemo treatment. According to Noel, my determination was still there as I made comments about him taking the long way to Brisbane from Hervey Bay by going through Nambour.

It may be difficult for other people to accept, as I do, that I reached a turning point in my illness during this time. I was suffering from hallucinations and two very pertinent things happened. The first was that I imagined I was standing on a pontoon which turned out to be a big turtle out in the ocean. I am not a swimmer but a voice was calling me to 'swim for it, Myra' and I was swimming, surrounded by small turtles bumping me in a particular direction. Then a voice called, 'the crocodiles are coming'. The voice kept repeating this. I was swimming and the little turtles were bumping me, apparently guiding me in the right direction. I feel this was a voice urging me to fight as I was at the peak of the crisis of my illness.

The second was that I imagined myself struggling with fishing line which was tangled around my hands and feet. My niece and two children were visiting me and I asked her and the children to help get it off. She tried to explain that there was no fishing line on me. Our minister, Jack Knapp, came in at this stage and my niece explained what was happening. Jack Knapp held me and comforted me and quietly went through the motions of untying the line from my hands and feet, talking to me all the time and explaining what he was doing. He then took the imaginary line out and threw it away. I felt at ease then and free of being tied down.

This was another indication of how faith and the kindness and help of others can affect our mind and, therefore, our body. I had responded to my fighting spirit and the help of others and passed the crisis that night, as the doctor told Noel. I truthfully believe that this is what happened.

This was the turning point of my illness. I was given five units of blood and since then I haven't looked back. I began to improve gradually and with the continued help of prayer, my husband, family and friends, I am now able to lead a practically normal life, continuing my chemo every six weeks in Brisbane.

This story of my recovery would not have happened without the wonderful support of my neighbours and particularly the care and comfort I received from our minister, Jack Knapp. I am the youngest of ten children and all my brothers and sisters are still alive. I have received great attention and support from them and their families.

I have had a few games of golf, I fish often, I drive myself to town or to visit and live as normally as possible. Cancer is not the end of the line. Your own determination, supported by prayer and all the people around you who care, makes it possible to fight back and not give in to our worst fears. One of the most important things I have found is to keep myself active. I love to crochet and knit and always have some piece of work under way. I pick it up when I sit down for a little rest or while watching TV. I find keeping my mind occupied relaxes me and there is no room for negative thoughts.

There is life with cancer and it is there to be lived, not to hide away. This attitude and the knowledge that it can be done with faith in our doctors and all those who help, and the good Lord who has guided them means life can still be sweet.

■ ■ ■

Choices?

'Riddled with cancer',
the doctor said.
'You can stay here
in hospital
or go home
and wait
for death!'

But I determined,
with help from
God
and help from
friends,
to seek another
way;
another possibility.

My journey
has taken me
through therapy
and dreams
and love of friends
and presence of church
and God,
to life, lived
with joy.

■ ■ ■

The Lord is my shepherd; I shall want nothing.
He makes me lie down in green pastures,
and leads me beside the waters of peace;
he renews life within me,
and for his name's sake guides me in the right path.
Even though I walk through a valley dark as death
I fear no evil, for thou art with me,
thy staff and thy crook are my comfort.

Psalm 23:1-4 (*New English Bible*)

■ ■ ■

Prayer

**God of darkness and of light,
whether life is obscure and painful
or whether it is bright and joyful,
keep me in your presence.**

Susan

> Frequently – as it did for Susan – discovering that we have cancer propels us into a different world. In this world, we may find pain and suffering, fear and uncertainty. We may also find courage and love and new friendships.
>
> It seems also that the things we normally tend to overlook take on a clarity which compels us to take notice. The brightness of the sun, the wetness of the rain, the caress of the wind, the song of birds, offer us a different way of looking at life. Things that once demanded our attention become rather insignificant and new insights are possible.

Walk briefly with Susan and look through her window. The last eight months have opened a window on a world I'd never seen first hand – that of the 'seriously ill'. It's a world where you listen intently to what other patients say; you watch their demeanour and accept people for what they are... (you are after all – *alive*); you meet people from all walks of life – all ages – you have a common bond. *You have cancer.*

My cancer resulted in a radical hysterectomy. I had a malignant tumour of the right ovary (it was the size of a baby's head). I have undergone a course of eight chemotherapy treatments every three weeks since my surgery in late November. A CAT scan in June gave me a clean bill of health. Throughout my treatment I always regarded myself as having *had* cancer. Surgery rid me of that intruder. I remember visualising this invader – a martian from some unknown land. How dare it inhabit my body!

This world I've entered beckons me to keep moving forward. Eight months on, I still have much work to do – as each day unravels, a greater insight into 'living' unfolds. It's a journey I need to take – I feel there's a pot of gold awaiting – (not gold coin but something more enduring – an inner peace that only adversity can determine). I feel I'm leading and those closest follow behind in their own time. Cancer didn't just strike me – it strikes family and friends together.

This new world was made so much easier with the help of my mother who nursed me through those treatments – good home cooking and plenty of rest together with the positive attitude that I would be right. My treatment was an insurance policy – just to make sure all cancer cells had been knocked out. I've since met people who haven't been as fortunate. I look searchingly into their beings to see how they cope. These brave souls really inspire you with their courage. Faith and hope propel them forward to face another day. None of us do this entirely on our own; the intertwining network of people in our lives all act like links in a chain.

Daily living can be a grind; it can demean. Negative pictures rear their ugly heads at each turn. Regaining your health cuts a swathe through this quagmire. You centre on the positive, see only the good and discard the trivia. Look around you; there is a wonderful world out there. Have you ever heard the orchestra played by suburban birds on a summer's morning? The morning after I came out of hospital, I was serenaded by this magical sound. It was truly thrilling. The last eight months have given me time to unwind. By slowing down the pace of life, you have time to recapture your dreams.

My life to date has not followed the fairy tale that is painted for us all in youth. Somehow it doesn't seem to matter now. My life is based squarely in reality. It's a *now* life; one based on days and what each day brings. I assure you I'm content. In another eight months, I'll be brimming over with the joy of *living*. I'll see you there.

■■■

Windows

I looked
through a window
and discovered
a new world
where,
each day
as life moves on,
my journey
leads me towards
that inner place
where stillness and peace
abide.

As I travel
I find,
surrounded by
the love
and courage
of others,
my path is blessed
with joy.

■■■

How blest are you who are in need;
the kingdom of God is yours.
How blest are you who now go hungry;
your hunger shall be satisfied.
How blest are you who weep now;
you shall laugh.

Luke 6:20-21 (*New English Bible*)

■■■

Prayer

Singing God,
thank you for life rediscovered,
for love, for the links that bind us together,
for the songs of birds,
for joy in living.

Bob

> Bob speaks of new awareness, of a wonderful life, of a wonderful family. He speaks of God tapping him on the shoulder and inviting him to look around at his life.
>
> Life itself is a growing in knowledge, understanding and wisdom. This does not usually happen, however as a slow steady progress but rather in bursts of insight flowing from particular events.
>
> When confronted by cancer and their own mortality, some people are angry that this should happen to them. Bob says he has never been angry over his illness. Rather, he treasures it as a gift which has given him time and incentive to reflect on his life and search for answers to the meaning of life.
>
> Bob draws out the difference for him between sudden death in which he would have no time for reflection and righting wrongs, and the slower process which has given him time to 'heal old wounds' and to learn 'to live a day at a time'.
>
> Bob's story suggests that he has discovered some wisdom. Perhaps you also, as you live through your own story, will gather wisdom

An important benefit for me in having cancer is the revelation to me of just how fortunate I am and what a fortunate life I've had. People have said to me in the past, 'You are lucky, you have done alright for yourself'. I've taken this for granted. Now I am facing, not so much my mortality as the sudden awareness of all the love that is around me. I had no need for the spiritual side but now that has become very important to me.

As I said, I've taken so many things for granted. If things weren't going right I'd get terribly despondent, particularly on the emotional side and I've said I would rather be dead than have to put up with this. I've realised how sinful that is because there are times when I really meant it. I no longer have that attitude because I've learned how wonderful life is. I'm seeing life through different eyes. Because of that, I can't help but appreciate what's happened to me. I have to appreciate that. It doesn't mean to say I'm glad I've got cancer and I'm glad I'm going to die. I've got to die of something.

It's as though God is talking to me. It really is. He's tapped me on the shoulder and said, 'Hey, come on. Just think about all this. Look around you and see what you've done; see what I've given you'. And I have. I've had a fortunate life. I must have been one of the chosen ones really. I think so. I've got three children and I can say my son is a fine man and a devoted father. I have two daughters who are devoted parents. They are both fine people.

If I can pass into the next life and say I've left behind three children and they are fine people that is one of the greatest gifts. As for my life, it's been a dream run, materially and in job satisfaction. I have a great wife who has stuck by me through thick and thin. We've had some battles but who hasn't.

Question. You've no sense of anger at having got this cancer?

None whatsoever! When I was told I had cancer it was almost like relief and I think that goes back to my wishing I was dead and I wasn't surprised because I had always suspected this would happen. No I'm not angry. How could I be angry? It gave me the biggest kick in the butt that I needed and reversed my thinking.

This life is wonderful. I've got no need to complain. I've got no need to want to die and every reason to want to live. It stirred the spiritual side of me and it has made me start to search for and find answers. I haven't found them all yet but have found a lot. No, I was not angry, am not angry, will never be angry! I'm sixty-three years old and have had a great life. What do I expect, how greedy can you get?

> *Question.* You say you are not angry about having cancer and maybe dying, yet you talk about wanting to live. How do you see that?

I believe that I will die when I am ready to die and when I am ready to die will be when God has told me I'm ready to die. He has said, 'OK, now you know'. I could have had a car accident driving home – bang – gone – and would not have had the opportunity to reflect as I have been able to reflect. I would not have had the opportunity to search as I have searched. I would not have been given the answers I have been given. I believe I am still to be given some more. I would not have had the opportunity – and this is very important – to heal some old wounds. It is terribly important to be able to do that. I think I can now die knowing that with all those whom I have wronged (that I've been able to get in touch with), outstanding matters have been put to rest. How lucky am I! It's because I am going to die of cancer that I've been given this opportunity. Heart attack – boom – you're gone!

> *Question.* There is a sense in which the cancer you have could be seen as a gift?

Absolutely. Beforehand, if I had been asked how I wanted to die, car accident, heart attack, quickly, or die with cancer struggling to survive for years, I'd have said give me the heart attack, give me the car accident. I would now say, give me what I've got. The end may be unpleasant. I don't know what it is going to be but with God's help I'll handle that. That's the way I see it. Yes, it been a gift, another gift.

> *Question.* So at the moment you are in the process of unwrapping the gift as it were?

Very much so. People like you – many little things – lead me along the way. There is a lovely nurse in the ward who lent me a book. Through that she really opened my eyes. I have an entirely different viewpoint on who God is and who I am, which is wonderful. I'll fight to live as long as I can because life is wonderful. Nobody has the right to wish they were dead.

For the first time in my life, I've learned to live a day at a time. I really couldn't understand previously the concept of living one day at a time. I used to think about tomorrow and live for tomorrow – ten years – twenty years planning for life into my eighties.

I found that it doesn't matter what I do. God's going to make the big decision not me. I've only got to look around me and the love that I've always had there from my family and I've known I've had it but it's different now. I receive it so gratefully and it humbles me, whereas before I just expected it. I've found love from ordinary people, people I've not known before; nice people. It overwhelms me, It makes me feel wonderful deep in my chest. When I die, I'll have that wonderful feeling with me. How could I be angry?

■ ■ ■

Awareness

New feelings
have come to life in me.
God
has given me time
to heal old wounds,
to forgive
and be forgiven

Today I speak
of love
and tolerance,
of peace
and God,
and know their meaning.

■■■

Make thy paths known to me, O Lord;
teach me thy ways.
Lead me in the truth and teach me;
thou art God my saviour.
For thee I have waited all the day long
for the coming of thy goodness, Lord.
Remember, Lord, thy tender care and thy love
unfailing,
shown from ages past.
Do not remember the sins and offences of my youth,
but remember me in thy unfailing love.
Psalm 25:4-7 (New English Bible)

■■■

Prayer

**God of wisdom,
you have given me the time for heart healing.
As I live towards my dying,
continue the healing in me
and give me joy in growing wisdom.**

Betty

Having to enter hospital for an operation, whether large or small, can leave many problems unresolved at home. When that is compounded by age, the need to care for another and the knowledge that the operation is because of cancer, the overall result can be traumatic. In some ways, some of the problems were solved for Betty by her husband also having to enter hospital.

Recovering in hospital, Betty recognised that, despite her current worries and fear of cancer, she could count many blessings. A loving husband and family had all contributed to these blessings.

When our perceptions are sharpened by serious illness, we all may find that there are many who care for us and show us concern.

Betty writes of an awareness of a presence which gave her comfort and peace. Perhaps you also have had this same sense of a presence. We may not be able to name this presence and perhaps this does not matter. What may be more important is that some thing comes to us and knows our name. It is as if we are then held in the palm of God's hand.

When I was diagnosed as having breast cancer, necessitating a partial mastectomy, I was in my seventies and preoccupied with caring for my husband (also in his seventies) who was nursing a fractured thigh. The bone refused to unite because of the presence of Pagets Disease and his only forms of locomotion were crutches and a wheelchair. My first reaction, therefore, to my trouble was mainly concern about how he could manage during my absence in hospital. I felt almost blameworthy to think I had caused a further complication for the family by developing cancer at such an inopportune time.

I tried to plan with our daughters just how we would manage. As it turned out, a few days after I went to hospital, my husband was admitted also. I think this eased the situation for our daughters in so far as they were able to see us both when visiting the hospital and so 'keep an eye on us'. I am sure, too, that it helped my recovery to be able to go down to the next floor to visit him.

It was not until I was in hospital that I was able to consider my illness. I had cancer and I had to come to grips with that fact. I realised that, like the majority of women, I feared breast cancer and did not under-estimate its threatening possibilities. I realised also that, whilst it could be disastrous to be stricken at any age by the disease, in my case I felt overwhelming gratitude that it had not developed earlier in my life.

My husband and I had enjoyed a wonderful life together and I had been there to care for him and give him practical support when needed. I had tried to help my children when they were growing up. I had been spared to see them grow into fine young women with much to contribute to life and their fellow beings. Every time they came to see me in hospital, I realised afresh how blessed I was to have them.

I had faith and a strong trust that all would be well. This attitude was fostered by my doctor who heeded my request to know exactly what had to be done. He drew diagrams to illustrate the procedure and even told me the position I would be placed in on the operating table. This did much to dispel my fear of the unknown.

Prior to this experience, I had never had a general anaesthetic nor any kind of surgery, nor had I been in hospital for more than a few days for the birth of each child. A new field of experience lay ahead. Would I be capable of exploring it?

As I lay in bed, with my body at rest, my perception sharpened, I became more receptive to surroundings and especially to the people about me: nurses, doctors, other patients, hospital visitors, domestic staff, the paper boy and the volunteers who looked after the flowers and operated the small mobile shop.

Central to everybody and everything and like a protective umbrella over us all was the pastoral care of the chaplains. This care was untiring and unstinted. The hospital motto, 'Not to be ministered unto but to minister', permeated all ranks within the hospital complex. This cumulative effect of care and concern was a gift, given to me as the result of my brush with cancer. For a few weeks I had lived in a world which, despite the different human personalities involved, exhibited no overt hatred, enmity, ill-humour, rejection, scorn or many of the attitudes which plague us. It was the way our world could be if we all tried harder.

A few nights after surgery, I was lying awake. I looked at my clock and saw that it was 8.45 p.m. I had some pain, but sleeplessness does not worry me unduly and I thought how quiet and peaceful the dark room was with just a finger of light from the corridor pointing into it. As I lay there, the feeling of peace persisted and slowly I became aware of a pervasive presence just above me. It hovered like a rectangle of soft grey cloud and seemed to be suspended over my left side at the site of the operation. I felt a surge of well-being, the cessation of pain and a most delightful soothing happiness which stayed with me for days.

Was I hallucinating? At that stage, I was not taking any new medications, only the ones I had been taking for years. Some weeks after leaving hospital, I learned that the Prayer Group from our church had their meeting on that particular night and my name had been on their list of those for whom they were offering prayers. It makes me very humble and grateful that they did this for me. Whatever the explanation of this experience, I regard it as a second gift from my brush with cancer.

■■■

One night

Hospitalisation!
Operation!
Fear and worry!
How would those at home
manage?

Then
one night,
in darkness and quietness,
I became aware
of your presence,
Lord,
and felt your
healing hand.

In answer to my prayers
and the prayers of others,
you came to me
as gracious gift.

■■■

O Lord, my heart is not proud,
nor are my eyes haughty;
I do not busy myself with great matters
or things too marvellous for me.
No; I submit myself, I account myself lowly,
as a weaned child clinging to its mother.
Psalm 131 (New English Bible)

■■■

Prayer

God of fear and worries,
you know me and have named me.
Touch my pain and still my fears
that I may know you deep within and find healing.

Ken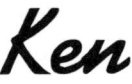

> Life appears to all of us to be never ending. While we all acknowledge that eventually we will die, that time seems always to be far off. When we are given the sort of news that Ken was given, time seems to shrink rather rapidly.
>
> In Australia, we are all fortunate to have skilled surgeons available and medical procedures to follow. This offers us considerable opportunity for healing or even a cure of our ills.
>
> Just as important is the support of people who are close to us and I expect we all experience this from time to time. This support, whether in prayer or in good wishes or in good deeds, is a powerful medicine in itself. We might all live longer if we were able to share our feelings more readily with each other.

I had a small lump on the side of my right eye and thought little of it until a visit to the specialist who said, 'I will operate on you the day after tomorrow at 1 o'clock. It will be a delicate operation to remove your saliva gland and a nerve and then do a skin graft on the eye, also a neck dissection'.

I thought this would never happen to me as there had never been any previous cases in my family and I was always confident of living to at least eighty-six years of age as my father had done before me.

After a five hour operation and during three days in intensive care, my thoughts were not very cheery, especially when I was told that at least thirty doses of radiotherapy would be needed at Peter MacCallum hospital.

I told myself I had to survive long enough to get home and get my affairs in order and finish all the unfinished jobs that were always going to be done 'some time'.

Prayer from my church, family and friends and the faith I had, helped me through this time of treatment and recuperation. Now I live from day to day, wondering how long the future holds for me, although it appears I am on the way to recovery and perhaps I will reach that eighty-six years of age.

■■■

86 years

My goal for life
is to live,
as my father did before me,
for 86 years.

The doctor said,
'In two days
I will operate
and follow that with
radiotherapy –
for thirty days.'

Has 86 years
I thought, become
a mere thirty days?

Whether thirty days
or thirty months
or thirty years,
be with me Lord
in friend and loved ones,
that I may hold your hand
and find peace.

■■■

...thou hast been my help,
and in the shadow of thy wings I
sing for joy.
My soul clings to thee;
thy right hand upholds me.
>> Psalm 63:7-8 (*Revised Standard Version of the Bible*)

■■■

Prayer

**God of days and years,
you have been with me until now.
Keep me in the palm of your hand
through the days and years that remain.**

Epilogue

The stories you have read are only a few of the multitude of stories that could be told. They are stories of pain and worry, of endurance and fortitude, but, more importantly, they are stories of hope.

Some are stories of faith and express the writers' strong conviction of God's presence with them.

Housewives, trades people, ministers, business people and professionals have contributed their stories to enable this book to be produced, in the hope that others might find strength and a sense of healing in sharing them.

Some of the contributors have died; others continue to live each day gladly. All of them have or had a strong conviction that life is to be lived now, not in the future, not in the past.

I hope you find healing even though you may not be cured. Looking for a cure can be difficult and demanding, requiring considerable commitment in dealing with the pain and disappointments. Those of us who have not experienced cancer can only walk alongside.

What we can all do, however, is find ways of getting in touch with the still centre of our life, the place where the Spirit dwells, and, encouraged by our sojourn there, continue in life each day. In this way, we may find healing.

I hope the stories in this book have opened windows for you through which you can look into yourself, and out to the world.